Don't Panic
Anxiety, Phobias & Tension

By Dr Andrew Page

ABOUT THE AUTHOR

Andrew Page is Associate Professor and Director of Clinical Psychology Training at the School of Psychology, University of Western Australia. He is also a consultant to one of Australia's premier private psychiatric hospitals, Perth Clinic, and is Co-Director of the Robin Winkler Clinic at the University of Western Australia. He has also worked as a clinical psychologist with the Clinical Research Unit for Anxiety and Depression, St Vincent's Hospital, Sydney.

He is the inaugural winner of the Tracy Goodall Early Career Award in recognition of innovation in research and treatment in cognitive and behaviour therapy and is past national president of the Australian Association for Cognitive and Behaviour Therapy.

He has written six books and numerous journal articles, chiefly on anxiety and its disorders.

CONTENTS

don't panic

ACKNOWLEDGEMENTS

Dedication
Cindy, Sarah, James and Joshua

Australian Women's Weekly Health Series
is published jointly by
ACP Publishing Pty Ltd (ABN 18 053 273 546) and
Media 21 Publishing Pty Ltd (ABN 82 090 635 073).
Editorial director ACP Books Susan Tomnay
Editorial directors Media 21 Philip Gore, Craig Osment
Marketing director Media 21 Stephen Balme

Produced by Media 21 Publishing,
30 Bay Street, Double Bay, NSW 2028.
Tel: (02) 9362 1800 Email: m21@media21.com.au
ACP Books GPO Box 4088, Sydney, NSW 2000
Tel: (02) 9282 8618 Email: acpbooks@acp.com.au

Publishing Manager (Sales) Jennifer McDonald
Publishing Manager (Rights & new projects) Jane Hazell
Business Manager Sally Lees

ACP Chief executive officer John Alexander
ACP Group Publisher Jill Baker **ACP Books Publisher** Sue Wannan

Printed by McPhersons Printing Group
Distribution Simon & Schuster. Tel: (02) 9415 9900

National Library of Australia Cataloguing-in-Publication entry
Page, Andrew, 1964- .
Don't panic : anxiety, phobias and tension : your four step program to
control anxiety disorder.
Rev. ed. Includes index.
ISBN 1 876624 87 6.
1. Anxiety. 2. Neuroses – Treatment. 3. Stress management.
I. Title. (Series : Australian women's weekly health series).
616.8522

don't panic

INTRODUCTION

Many people suffer from anxiety, but far, far too many suffer from panics and fears, continual worry and troubling thoughts, to the point where the comfort and peace of their lives is disturbed. Some people with worries and panics will require professional help to recover, but there is much that you can do to manage your own anxiety well. The first step is understanding the meaning of the symptoms and the second is knowing how to cope with them.

This book will teach both things. Dr Page is a very experienced clinical psychologist. He has treated many people with severe anxiety disorders and understands just how terrible they can feel. Most importantly, he is able to give his advice in simple, straightforward language that makes it easy for everyone to understand and benefit. If you suffer from anxiety, you should buy this book. Then do just what it says!

Professor Gavin Andrews MD
St Vincent's Hospital
Sydney

CHAPTER 1

ANXIETY
KNOW YOUR ENEMY

Anxiety is a normal human emotion. But for one out of every 10 people, anxiety prevents them carrying out everyday activities. Such problem anxiety may take four different forms:

- Spontaneous attacks of panic
- Excessive fears about situations that most people handle with ease
- Uncontrollable worries
- Excessive physical tension

In each case, anxiety is too high. It is anxiety that has taken control.

The first step in overcoming problem anxiety is to know your enemy. You must recognise the

> **The first step in overcoming problem anxiety is to know your enemy.**

forms in which problem anxiety presents itself. Let's take a quick look at each of these now. We'll cover them in more detail in later chapters, and give you strategies for overcoming them.

WHAT IS PANIC?

Panic occurs when anxiety rapidly reaches a peak in situations where most people would not feel anxious. The panic appears "out of the blue". As a result, sufferers not only feel frightened,

don't panic

but may also be puzzled about the origin of their sensations and expect the worst. During panic, you may experience:

- Intense fear
- Breathlessness
- Choking or smothering
- Tingling in your hands or feet
- Pounding heart
- Faintness
- Pressure, tightness, or pain in the chest
- Trembling or shaking
- Dizziness or lightheadedness
- Hot or cold flushes
- Dry mouth
- Nausea or "butterflies"
- "Jelly legs"
- Blurred vision or spots before the eyes
- Muscle tension

You may think:
- I might be dying
- I might lose control, embarrass myself and others will see
- I might be going mad or crazy
- I might hurt myself or others
- I might collapse and pass out

You may try to:
- Flee from the situation
- Distract yourself
- Get help or reassurance

FEAR OF FEAR ITSELF

Attacks of panic are common to anxiety problems. Sometimes they are spontaneous, taking you by surprise. At other times, they occur in predictable situations. Either way, the attack is terrifying.

It is therefore no surprise that you come to fear the occurrence of fear itself. "Fear of fear" varies from person to person. Usually people

> **Usually people attempt to avoid places where panic is likely or help unavailable.**

attempt to avoid places where panic is likely or where help may be unavailable. When there is no avoidance, yet frequent or feared attacks of spontaneous panic occur, this is called panic disorder. More about panic, and how to master it, in Chapters 3 and 4.

PHOBIC FEARS

Many individuals who have attacks of panic cannot continue their daily routine. They structure their lives so that anxiety and its effects are minimised.

Some avoid situations in which panic occurs (such as shopping centres, bank queues, public transport) hoping that fear will decrease. Others seek the help of doctors, friends, relatives, or even complete strangers, fearing that they may collapse, die, lose control, or go crazy.

When these avoidances restrict daily life, then you are said to have agoraphobia, a term that combines two Greek words – "agora" meaning "market place" and "phobia" meaning "fear" – and is often mistakenly understood as an excessive fear of open spaces.

For other people, attacks of panic occur at predictable times and places. People who experience panic under the scrutiny of others

don't panic

may have a social phobia or social anxiety disorder. Typical situations feared when you have a social anxiety disorder include:

- Public speaking
- Eating and drinking in front of others
- Writing or signing your name in public
- Meeting new people
- Participating in groups
- Using pubic toilets

Other predictable places where panics occur include heights, enclosed places, the dark, water and aeroplanes. Panic may also occur in the presence of small animals, insects, spiders and reptiles. When such fears become excessive and interfere with your life, you may be suffering from a specific phobia.

Fearful avoidance can also occur in the form of compulsive behaviour. Compulsions happen when you feel compelled to act in a precise way,

Obsessions burst again and again into your consciousness, despite yourself.

often checking the same thing over and over again, or washing and cleaning over and over again. Very often these compulsions are performed in response to an obsession.

Obsessions are distressing thoughts, mental images, or impulses that burst again and again into your consciousness, despite your best attempts to keep them out of mind.

When such checking, washing, or obsessional thoughts interfere with a person's life, it is called obsessive compulsive disorder. Acting out your compulsions may seem to reduce anxiety, but the relief is only temporary – you're left feeling distressed and depressed in the short-term, and more anxious in the longer-term.

Chapter 6, on facing your fears, will be especially important in helping you to overcome phobic fears, obsessions and compulsions.

WORRY AND PHYSICAL TENSION

Anxiety also shows itself in the form of uncontrollable worry. Usually such worries centre on family, work, finances and illness. They intrude into your awareness and dominate your

> **Uncontrollable worries may leave you edgy, keyed up, and more likely to panic.**

thoughts. These worries lead to physical tension, leaving you apprehensive, edgy, keyed up, easily tired and more likely to panic. If uncontrollable worry and physical tension have persisted for months or years, you would be said to be suffering from generalised anxiety disorder.

OTHER WORRIES

Worry is part of other anxiety problems too. In these cases, worry tends to focus on particular problems or situations.

Someone with panic disorder may worry about panic attacks; someone with agoraphobia may worry about losing control in public; someone with social phobia may worry about the opinions of others; and someone with a specific phobia may worry about possible danger from spiders, snakes and so on; while the hallmark of generalised anxiety disorder is excessive worry about everyday concerns. Chapters 7 and 8, on straight thinking, will teach you how to master your worrying thoughts; Chapters 9 and 10 will be helpful in overcoming tension.

IS SOMETHING PHYSICALLY WRONG WITH ME?

Many physical problems have symptoms that resemble those of anxiety. If you think there may be something physically wrong with you it's sensible to discuss your concerns about your health with your doctor. A physical checkup and a full blood count will usually be conducted to rule out possible diseases.

It's wise to request these assessments, but remember, uncontrollable worry often revolves around (baseless) fear of illness. If you find yourself repeatedly having the same tests, and they are always negative, it is probably time to concentrate on managing the worrying thoughts.

FACT FILE

Summary
While anxiety problems can only be accurately diagnosed in consultation with a clinical psychologist, psychiatrist or your doctor, these four themes run through all such problems:
- *Spontaneous panic*
- *Phobias*
- *Uncontrollable worry*
- *Physical tension*

You will know which of these presents most difficulty for you. In the following chapters, we look at each in turn, and show you how to understand and master panic and phobic fears, as well as uncontrollable worries and excessive tension.

This four-step program will allow you to regain control over anxiety, restoring its role as a normal and useful emotion.

CHAPTER 2

ANXIETY
KNOW YOUR FRIEND

Not all anxiety causes problems. In fact, anxiety is a normal emotion that serves to protect you from danger. To see how anxiety develops into panic, phobias, uncontrollable worries and excessive tension, it is necessary to understand normal anxiety.

Anxiety is an automatic alarm response with a number of important advantages for you.

YOUR AUTOMATIC ALARM RESPONSE

Imagine yourself turning a street corner and coming face to face with a very large dog. It looks at you, snarls, barks and then starts to run towards you. Your brain automatically becomes aware of danger. Adrenaline is immediately released to activate your involuntary nervous system. This activation – called the flight or fight response – causes a set of bodily changes (see opposite). These changes enable you to act quickly, avoid injury and escape danger.

• Breathing speeds up and the nostrils and lungs open wide, increasing the amount of oxygen available to the muscles.

• Heart rate and blood pressure increase so that the oxygen and nutrients required by your body's cells can be transported quickly to where they are needed.

THE FLIGHT OR FIGHT RESPONSE

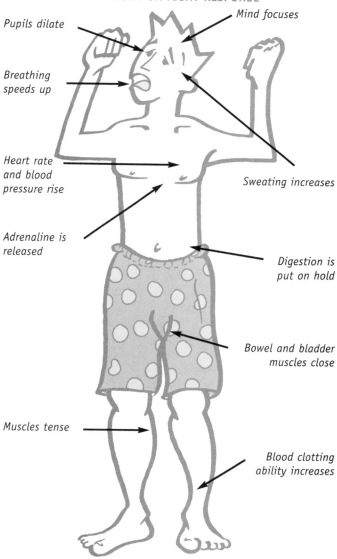

Pupils dilate

Mind focuses

Breathing speeds up

Heart rate and blood pressure rise

Sweating increases

Adrenaline is released

Digestion is put on hold

Bowel and bladder muscles close

Muscles tense

Blood clotting ability increases

don't panic

• Blood is diverted to muscles, particularly the large leg muscles to allow you to run away. Less blood is sent to areas that do not immediately need nutrition. Blood moves away from your face and you may turn "pale with fright".

• Muscles become instantly tense, preparing you to react quickly.

• Blood clotting ability increases in order to minimise blood loss should injury occur.

Your mind becomes focused, preoccupied with the thought: 'What is the danger?'

• Sweating increases to cool your body, stopping it overheating when strenuous physical activity begins. Blood vessels expand and move towards the skin to cool the blood. This may show as blushing or blotchy skin.

• Your mind becomes focused, preoccupied with the thought: "What is the danger and how can I get to safety?"

• Digestion is put on hold. While running from a dog it is not important to digest your most recent meal, so the stomach goes on strike. Your mouth dries up as less saliva is made. Food sits heavily in the stomach and you may feel nausea or "butterflies". Instead, glucose – a form of sugar that your body can use quickly – is released from your liver to provide energy.

• Your immune system slows down. In the short-term, your body puts all of its efforts into escaping. Who cares if you stopped yourself catching a cold if three seconds later you were attacked by a dog?

• Sphincter muscles of the bowel and bladder tighten so that no trail is left by which a predator could track you down.

It is the automatic triggering of this "flight or fight" response that allows you to run and escape. The flight or fight response is an automatic reaction that will prepare you to fly from danger. Only when escape is impossible will you turn and fight for your life.

Not all anxiety is of the same intensity. The thought of an examination or a job interview may raise your anxiety but not usually to the same degree as when you're faced with a vicious dog. But whatever the degree of anxiety felt, it is controlled by the involuntary nervous system. The flight or fight response is triggered by vague worries, just as it is by full-blown panic. In each case the alarm goes off, but to a lesser or greater degree.

I'm afraid I'll wet or soil myself
Many people feel the urge to release bowel or bladder when anxious. However, the chance of this actually happening is comfortingly low.

Most often, loss of bowel or bladder control occurs when people are trapped in terrifying situations for very long periods. An example would be a soldier stuck in a trench, waiting for the enemy to drop a bomb on him.

Even the longest panic attacks don't cause loss of control because the overriding desire is to escape. As we've seen, when preparing to flee, the body makes every effort to stop you leaving any evidence by which a predator may pursue you.

FALSE ALARMS

Unfortunately, some alarms are false alarms. You just have to walk past some parked cars and their alarms go off. Although you aren't trying to steal the car, the alarm still reacts as though you're a thief. The problem is that the alarm is

don't panic

too sensitive. In the same way, anxiety problems start when the flight or fight response is too sensitive. When the alarm is too sensitive, the response is triggered at the wrong times.

If your anxiety alarm goes off too easily, you will be more likely to become anxious in situations where others would not feel anxious. Consider the following people's experiences:

- Mary, 31, has agoraphobia. Standing in a shopping queue, she felt dizzy, lightheaded, and slightly "unreal". Having an easily-triggered

Dizzy, lightheaded and slightly 'unreal' – results of an over-sensitive alarm reaction.

alarm reaction, she thought: "What if I go crazy and I run amok – shouting, swearing, and hitting people?" She left the shop immediately, retreating to the safety of her home.

- William, 27, has social anxiety disorder. As the automatic teller was out of order, he went to make a withdrawal from a bank. His flight or fight response was triggered when he noticed his hand shaking and he thought: "What if my signature is unreadable? The teller will call the manager to watch me sign my name again. I will shake so much they will think I am using someone else's account and call the police." Feeling panicky, William left to look for another automatic teller.

- Joan, 45, has generalised anxiety disorder. Her anxiety alarm was triggered while hearing about her country's economic difficulties.

She thought: "What if I lose my job and my husband cannot find work? We will not be able to pay our mortgage, the house will be repossessed and we will be homeless!" Joan spent a tense evening and a sleepless night worrying about as-yet non-existent problems.

• Dale, 19, has a specific phobia of enclosed spaces. Her flight or fight response was activated when she entered the fire stairs. Having already decided that the lift was too dangerous, she thought: "What if all the doors are locked and I am trapped in here for ever?" She ran down the stairs and discovered, with great relief, that the exit was unlocked.

• Maria, 25, has obsessive-compulsive disorder. Her flight or fight response is triggered when she has thoughts like: "Oh no, what if I've left the stove on and the house burns down." She then returns to the stove and checks seven

Panic, fear, worry and tension: all can occur where others may not feel anxious.

times that each knob is placed in the "off" position and passes her hand seven times over each hot plate to check that it is cold.

Each one of these people experienced significant amounts of panic, fear, worry and tension in situations that would not cause anxiety in others. The alarm reaction, made to protect them from fierce dogs and other physical dangers, was triggered at the wrong time, by an inappropriate stimulus.

The simple answer is because your anxiety alarm is too sensitive. Just why it has become so sensitive is a more complex question.

Psychological research has revealed three causes of an over-sensitive anxiety alarm: stress, inheritance and overbreathing.

Stress

Stressful life events may be physical (such as illness, childbirth, or overwork) or psychological (such as financial worries, daily hassles, or family

> **If one or both of your parents are anxious, chances are that you may be too.**

difficulties). Whether physical or psychological, stressful life events make you uptight.

The involuntary nervous system becomes more activated, so panic, worries and tension are triggered more easily.

Inheritance

Many people with anxiety problems see themselves as "nervous" people. Nervousness is an inherited personality characteristic. If one or both of your parents are anxious, chances are that you, too, may be generally anxious, and more likely to see threats in otherwise safe objects and situations.

Some objects and situations are more threatening than others, and the tendency to fear these is also something we inherit. They include heights, confined spaces, strangers, reptiles, spiders, insects, blood and injury. All of these objects and situations would have been dangers to our ancient ancestors, who lived a very different life from ours. Although we all inherit a tendency to become alarmed by such dangers, for some people this normal alarm is too sensitive – and so phobias develop.

Overbreathing

Breathing too much or too deeply is one of the more subtle of the causes of anxiety. Because of its central role in the escalation of anxiety, overbreathing will be discussed fully in the next chapter.

FACT FILE

Summary
The flight or fight response is an alarm reaction that allocates the body's resources to protect you from danger. If you have anxiety problems, this normal alarm reaction is over-sensitive.

Here, it is enough to say that overbreathing is a part of the flight or fight response that makes your anxiety alarm more sensitive.

CHAPTER 3

ALL ABOUT
PANIC

Panic involves the lightning-fast escalation of anxiety into terror. As mentioned in the previous chapter, one of the ways to escalate anxiety into panic is overbreathing. Faster and deeper breathing is a part of the flight or fight response. This rapidly increases levels of oxygen in the blood and decreases blood levels of carbon dioxide. Just as you would fill your petrol tank before a petrol strike, your body fills up with oxygen before you have to run from danger. As a result, when physical activity begins there is plenty of oxygen in reserve.

When overbreathing occurs without physical activity, anxiety escalates into panic. To see how overbreathing raises anxiety, it helps first to understand the mechanics of normal breathing.

NORMAL BREATHING

Your body is made up of millions of cells. To survive, cells require oxygen. Whenever you breathe in, oxygen is taken into the lungs. From there, it passes into tiny blood vessels surrounding the lungs. Once in the blood, the oxygen sticks to the red blood cells, enabling it to be carried around the body.

Later, the oxygen is released from the red blood cells and passes into the body's cells. Like

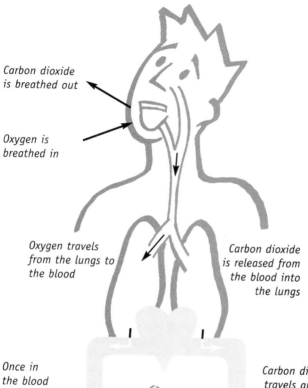

Carbon dioxide
is breathed out

Oxygen is
breathed in

Oxygen travels
from the lungs to
the blood

Carbon dioxide
is released from
the blood into
the lungs

Once in
the blood
the oxygen
sticks to
the red
blood cells

Carbon dioxide
travels around
the blood

Body's cells

Oxygen is released from
the red blood cells and
travels to the body's cells

The body's cells release
carbon dioxide into
the blood

don't panic

factories, these cells use raw materials (oxygen) and produce waste products (carbon dioxide). The carbon dioxide is then released into the blood, transported to the lungs, and breathed out.

How do the red blood cells know when to release the oxygen? The presence of carbon dioxide in the blood causes the red blood cells to release oxygen. Said another way, carbon dioxide makes the red blood cells less sticky and so the oxygen becomes unstuck.

For the body to work properly, therefore, there needs to be the right balance between oxygen and carbon dioxide. When these are balanced, anxiety does not escalate into panic.

HOW OVERBREATHING CAUSES PROBLEMS

Overbreathing which occurs as part of the flight or fight response brings about a short-lived imbalance between oxygen and carbon dioxide in the blood. Once physical flight or fight begins, oxygen is used up and carbon dioxide is produced, restoring balance to the blood.

If you do not flee or fight, the imbalance between oxygen and carbon dioxide remains for longer periods. The build-up of oxygen in the blood is not a cause for concern.

However, the drop in carbon dioxide causes problems. Although there is plenty of oxygen in the blood, it is not released from the red blood cells. Breathing out your carbon dioxide has made the red blood cells sticky for oxygen. Paradoxically, by breathing in more oxygen (and breathing out more carbon dioxide) you reduce the oxygen reaching the body's cells.

In addition, overbreathing has another important effect. Overbreathing causes the blood

don't panic

vessels to shrink. Consequently, the oxygen being released has to travel further from the blood to the cells. As a result, little oxygen reaches the cells of the body and brain.

These two effects – the decreased release of oxygen from the red blood cells and

Breathlessness is your brain's recognition that something is not quite right.

the shrinkage of blood vessels – produce a variety of sensations which, to the anxious person, sound all too familiar. The cells of the brain are reached by less oxygen, and so they begin to work less efficiently.

The drop in oxygen is slight and harmless, but it will be experienced in the following ways:
- Dizziness
- Lightheadedness
- Confusion
- Visual disturbance (for example, blurred vision)
- Feelings of unreality
- Breathlessness

Breathlessness is your brain's recognition that something is not quite right. As a result, you will breathe more heavily and deeply.

However, this strategy will make the situation worse, because you will breathe out even more carbon dioxide.

There is also a decrease in the amount of oxygen reaching the body's cells. You experience a variety of sensations associated with the decrease in oxygen. Common sensations include:
- Increased heart rate (to pump more blood around the body)

- Numbness and tingling in hands and feet
- Clammy hands
- Stiffness and shakiness in the muscles
- "Jelly legs"

As well as the direct effects of overbreathing, there are a number of indirect effects. Since overbreathing is hard physical work, you may feel

> **Since overbreathing is hard physical work, you may feel hot, flushed and sweaty.**

hot, flushed, and sweaty; not to mention tired and exhausted. And since you're also taking quick, short breaths from the chest, the muscles become tired, leading to chest pain and tightness. In addition, overbreathing causes saliva to evaporate, leaving your mouth dry.

If overbreathing keeps going, the body changes strategy. Until now it has been encouraging you to breathe faster and harder.

Now it attempts to slow your breathing down to increase the level of carbon dioxide in the blood. For example, your throat will tighten to reduce the amount of carbon dioxide breathed out and to reduce the amount of oxygen breathed in.

If successful, the build-up of carbon dioxide will allow the available oxygen to be released from the red blood cells.

During this second stage of overbreathing, you will experience the body's efforts as:

- Dizziness and nausea
- Choking or smothering (as the throat closes slightly)
- Temporary paralysis of some muscles
- Momentary blackouts

don't panic

OVERBREATHING WHEN ANXIOUS

If you remember what we said about the flight or fight response, you will see it overlaps with overbreathing. This is not surprising, given that increases in breathing are part of the flight or fight response. However, if you are already mildly anxious and begin to overbreathe it is clear that symptoms of anxiety will escalate rapidly. One thing leads to another:

- The increased heart rate associated with anxiety will escalate rapidly.
- The increased heart rate associated with anxiety will be made worse by overbreathing.
- The increased blood pressure will be raised further by constriction of the blood vessels ... and so on.

In addition, overbreathing is unpleasant and people may come to fear overbreathing itself. For some, the sensations are a source of anxiety. The racing heart or chest pain may be taken as signalling a heart attack or stroke. The feelings of unreality may be interpreted as signalling

The sensations are themselves a source of anxiety, perhaps signalling a breakdown.

a nervous breakdown. The dizziness and weak legs may signal that fainting is about to occur. The desire to flee may be thought to indicate loss of control.

For other people, the sensations contribute to anxiety. A person who is afraid of shaking in public will become anxious when the muscles tense and shake. Others, who fear that other people will think less of them if their anxiety is

don't panic

visible, may become afraid while blushing.
For most people, the increase in symptoms of anxiety brought about by overbreathing are distressing because of their rapid rise.

Many people worry that the anxiety may cause physical damage, that a nervous breakdown will occur, or that the unpleasant experience will continue forever. Yet, whatever interpretations are made about the sensations, it is clear that they are misinterpretations of normal physical changes due to overbreathing and the triggering of the flight or fight response.

THE VICIOUS CIRCLE OF ANXIETY AND OVERBREATHING

Once you become worried about the symptoms of overbreathing you enter a vicious circle. At the start of the vicious circle is a trigger – possibly a situation previously associated with anxiety, perhaps a bodily sensation (such as shaking, blushing, or heart palpitations).

Sometimes the trigger may be a memory of past anxiety. Other times it may be anticipation of a difficult situation. It may even be a thought that triggers the vicious circle: "No one else has thoughts like these," you may tell yourself, "I must be really strange, wicked or immoral."

Whatever the trigger, the situation is perceived as dangerous or threatening. You think: "Oh no. What if ... ?"

• Someone with panic disorder may think: "Oh no, my heart skipped a beat, what if I have a heart attack?"

• A person with agoraphobia may think: "Oh no, the only seat left in the cinema is in the middle, what if I need to escape quickly?"

THE VICIOUS CIRCLE OF OVERBREATHING

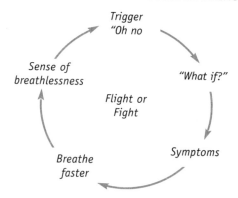

Trigger
"Oh no

"What if?"

Sense of
breathlessness

Flight or
Fight

Symptoms

Breathe
faster

- A person with social anxiety disorder may think: "Oh no, I am being watched, what if I make a mistake and everyone laughs at me?"
- Someone with generalised anxiety disorder may think: "Oh no, my child looks unwell, what if she has leukemia?"
- Someone with obsessive-compulsive disorder may think, "Oh no, what if I don't wash, something bad will happen and I'll be to blame."

Common to each of these thoughts is the fact that the situation is labelled as threatening or dangerous. As a result, the flight or fight response is triggered.

Part of this alarm involves overbreathing, but overbreathing in the absence of physical activity leads to increased anxiety. It does this because overbreathing leads to breathlessness which encourages faster breathing.

In turn, overbreathing and activation of the flight or fight response produce bodily and mental sensations. If you then worry about these sensations you end up in a vicious circle.

don't panic

FACT FILE

Summary

• *Overbreathing is a normal part of the flight or fight response.*

• *Overbreathing causes an imbalance between oxygen and carbon dioxide that decreases the oxygen reaching the body and brain. This in turn produces bodily and mental sensations that contribute to a rapid increase in anxiety.*

• *Overbreathing is not physically or mentally dangerous.*

Overbreathing is not life-threatening, however. Faster breathing is central to the flight or fight response. It is part of the body's normal alarm reaction to protect you from harm. Imagine a car alarm that caused the car to explode every time a burglar attempted to steal it. It would hardly be an effective protection. Likewise, a flight or fight response that caused a person to become permanently anxious, have a heart attack, lose control, go crazy, collapse or die would not be a very effective protection either.

Activation of the flight or fight response and the associated overbreathing are normal responses, both of which are designed to keep you safe and alive.

False alarms are intensely unpleasant and even incapacitating, but they are not dangerous.

don't panic

CHAPTER 4

SLOW BREATHING TO CONTROL PANIC

Overbreathing and its effects are quite subtle. In fact, most people who overbreathe are not aware that they are doing so. This is why you need to become aware of how and when you overbreathe. One clue that you overbreathe while worrying is frequent sighing or yawning.

Notice how often you sigh or yawn next time you talk about or approach what you fear. You breathe out a lot of carbon dioxide as you take larger breaths or sigh frequently.

If your breathing increases at such times, you will need to use slow breathing while you start to face your fears.

DO YOU *SOMETIMES* BREATHE TOO QUICKLY?

Overbreathing may occur as you anticipate doing something that makes you anxious.

During the anxious anticipation your breathing increases slightly, rising further as you get closer to what you fear.

Consequently, you enter the vicious circle of overbreathing (see previous chapter) and your anxiety spirals into panic.

DO YOU *ALWAYS* BREATHE TOO QUICKLY?

If you always breathe too quickly, you will take in too much oxygen and breathe out too much carbon dioxide. This creates an imbalance between oxygen and carbon dioxide that causes the effects of overbreathing to appear.

Usually this is just enough to leave you slightly apprehensive, perhaps even feeling dizzy and lightheaded.

CHECKING YOUR OWN BREATHING
To see if you are breathing too much, count how quickly you breathe right now.

- Count one breath in and out as "one"
- Count the next breath in and out as "two"

Continue counting this way until one minute has passed. You will probably find it difficult to count your normal breathing rate. As soon as you focus your attention on your breathing it feels faster or slower than normal. Don't worry. Try to get the best possible estimate of your normal breathing rate and write it below.

Number of breaths per minute: ____

The average person needs to take around 10-12 breaths per minute when relaxed. If you are breathing a lot faster while at rest you will definitely need to master the slow breathing described later in the chapter.

Before discussing slow breathing, let's consider situations that make overbreathing (and hence panic) more likely.

WHEN DO YOU OVERBREATHE?
Are you breathing through your mouth?
As the mouth is bigger than the nose it is much easier to overbreathe through your mouth. When possible, always breathe through your nose.

don't panic

Are you smoking too much?

Tobacco accelerates the fight or flight response. This is because nicotine releases adrenaline, one hormone that, as we've seen, activates this response. Also, carbon monoxide is breathed in while you smoke. Given a choice, red blood cells will select carbon monoxide, rather than oxygen,

The effects of smoking can make your anxiety more likely to spiral into panic.

to stick to them. This reduces the oxygen reaching your brain and body. Finally, nicotine causes blood vessels to shrink. This reduces the amount of oxygen reaching your body's cells.

All three effects make anxiety more likely to spiral into panic. Naturally, it is better not to smoke, but if this is not possible, do not smoke before entering a situation where you expect to have difficulty controlling anxiety.

Are you drinking too much tea or coffee?

For a significant number of people caffeine stimulates anxiety. Switch to decaffeinated coffee or very weak tea. If anxiety decreases when you cut out caffeine and increases again when you restart, it is best to avoid caffeine until you are confident about controlling anxiety.

Are you getting enough sleep?

Tiredness increases vulnerability to overbreathing and anxiety. Try to get to bed and get up at a regular time. If the problem of tiredness persists, you may wish to consult a clinical psychologist or your doctor to discuss possible non-drug or drug treatments.

don't panic

Are you suffering from premenstrual tension?

Premenstrual hormonal changes decrease blood levels of carbon dioxide, making overbreathing more noticeable. For this reason you may experience a worsening of panic-like sensations before menstruation. Once you have become aware of these changes, you will be able to use the techniques you are about to learn, to deal with premenstrual panic.

Do you rush?

Impatience is a sign of anxiety. Anxious people often race past everyone on the street, rush

Racing past people, rushing at work, always hurrying ... all signs of anxiety.

around at work and hurry to meet deadlines. The impatience that drives this frenzy comes from anxiety. If you slow down, you will become less impatient and feel less like rushing.

Do you overbreathe when anxious?

When the flight or fight response is triggered you breathe faster. This normal response prepares you for vigorous physical activity.

If you do not fight or flee, overbreathing occurs. As a result, anxiety rises quickly and becomes overwhelming.

It is obviously important to recognise overbreathing in these situations.

If overbreathing can be stopped, anxiety will not spiral into panic. If you think back to the previous chapter you will see that you will be able to stop the escalation into panic. You will be able to jump out of the vicious circle.

SLOW BREATHING TECHNIQUE

To break out of this circle, you need to do two things. First, you need to increase the level of carbon dioxide in the blood. This will allow the available oxygen to be released into the body's cells, slowly restoring you to normal.

To achieve this goal, at the first sign of anxiety, you should:

- Stop what you are doing and stay where you are. Do not flee!
- Hold your breath for 10 seconds. (Use a watch because time seems to go faster when anxious.) Do not take a deep breath.

Using a watch, hold your breath for 10 seconds. Breathe out and say, 'Relax.'

- After 10 seconds, breathe out and say the word "Relax" to yourself.

Secondly, you need to decrease your breathing rate. Doing so will keep oxygen and carbon dioxide in balance.

To achieve this goal, after you have breathed out, you should:

- Breathe in and out (through your nose) slowly in a six-second cycle. Breathe in for three seconds and out for three seconds, saying "Relax" to yourself on every breath out. This produces a breathing rate of 10 breaths per minute,
- At the end of each minute (after 10 breaths), hold your breath again for 10 seconds and then breathe on a six-second cycle.
- Continue breath-holding and slow breathing till symptoms of overbreathing have gone.

don't panic

YOUR DAILY BREATHING RATE RECORD

	8.00am		12 noon	
Date	Before	After	Before	A
Example	21	12	18	1

Because the slow breathing technique first restores and then maintains a balance between oxygen and carbon dioxide, it needs to be done at the first sign that anxiety is rising.

If you remember to act immediately and do these things at the first sign of overbreathing, anxiety will not spiral into panic.

The more you practise the slow breathing technique, the better you will become at using it to manage anxiety and panic.

Secondly, the more you practise, the slower your normal breathing rate will become.

6.00pm		9.00pm	
Before	After	Before	After
14	8	15	15

WHAT IF I FEEL WORSE?

A few people find that anxiety increases when they slow their breathing. These are usually people who have been overbreathing for a long time. The body has compensated for overbreathing and, when breathing slows down, an alarm reaction goes off. You will feel anxious, want to take large gulps of air, feel lightheaded, dizzy, and may even notice your heart racing.

These sensations are actually a sign of progress. You are retraining your involuntary nervous system to stop compensating for overbreathing. If it is a slow learner, be patient and work hard. Over time these sensations will decline. Keep a record of the intensity of the sensations every time you slow your breathing and you will see that indeed they are decreasing.

The most common mistakes that people make when controlling panic with slow breathing are that they start too late or finish too early.

If you finish too early, panic will return immediately you stop slow breathing. If you

'Flight or fight' may be an involuntary response. But you can control your panic.

start too late, the imbalance between oxygen and carbon dioxide takes a long time to restore.

Either way, you are likely to feel as if you are not making progress.

Remember, slow breathing is your way of controlling panic. Activation of the flight or fight response may be controlled by the involuntary nervous system, but breathing can also be controlled by the voluntary nervous system. Breathing therefore provides a way for you to take control over the flight or fight response and stop the spiral of anxiety into panic.

DAILY RECORD OF BREATHING RATE
Monitor your breathing at the times shown on the table on pages 34/35. Because your breathing rate will be higher while busy or exercising, practise slow breathing while resting.

• Count your normal breathing rate for one minute. On the first breath in and out, count "one"; on the next breath in and out count "two", and so on. Do not slow your breathing.

This will provide a "before" reading.

- Do your slow breathing practice. Hold your breath for 10 seconds and then breathe for one minute on a six-second cycle.
- Count your normal breathing rate again over one minute. This will give an "after" reading that you can write in the table.

As you complete the table, you will be able to check that by doing the exercise you are slowing your normal breathing rate.

You will also be able to see that with practice your "before" breathing rate slowly decreases to 10-12 breaths per minute.

FACT FILE

Summary
Breathing too quickly or deeply creates an imbalance between oxygen and carbon dioxide. The imbalance produces various sensations that cause anxiety to spiral into panic. You can control panic by slowing your breathing.

- *Hold your breath for 10 seconds.*
- *Breathe out and say "Relax" to yourself.*
- *Breathe in for about three seconds, and out for three seconds.*
- *Say "Relax" each time you breathe out.*
- *Repeat the cycle until panic goes away.*

STOP!
Now it is time to stop reading and master the art of slow breathing. Spend a minimum of four days practising so that it starts to become second nature. Until it becomes automatic, you will have difficulty doing others things (such as walking, speaking or driving) while controlling your breathing. You should also keep up the practice until uncomfortable feelings (resulting from your body's attempts to compensate for previous overbreathing) no longer occur.

don't panic

CHAPTER 5

ALL ABOUT PHOBIAS
AND COMPULSIONS

Now that you understand how slow breathing stops panic, it is time to face your fears. While you have probably tried to do this in the past, it is time to attempt it differently. You can use the slow breathing technique to control anxiety, stopping it spiralling into panic.

Although anxiety will still occur, facing your fears is essential. How will you ever be sure that you can control your anxiety until you confront it and win?

PHOBIC FEAR AND AVOIDANCE

A universal truth about anxiety is that avoidance makes fears worse. To understand why this is so, consider these three facts:

- Anxiety is unpleasant
- Avoiding fear-provoking situations or activities stops anxiety
- Escaping when anxiety is rising brings enormous relief

If you think about these facts you will see that not facing your fear is, at first sight, sensible. Who would deliberately make themselves more anxious?

Think about the situations that make you very anxious. For people with social anxiety disorder, these may include writing, eating and public speaking. For people with panic disorder and agoraphobia, these may include activities that increase panicky feelings (such as running and being in hot, humid conditions), or situations in which a panic may be thought to be dangerous, difficult or embarrassing (such as travelling by public transport, driving, shopping, standing in queues or sitting in the middle of a cinema).

For people with generalised anxiety disorder, phobic avoidances may include such things as avoiding watching the news, or seeking

What happens when you avoid what you fear? Don't you feel the 'reward' of relief?

reassurance from doctors whenever a pain is felt. For people with obsessive-compulsive disorder, the repeated washing and checking may reduce anxiety. There may be mental rituals (counting or repeating a phrase) that reduce anxiety.

Think about what happens to you when you avoid or escape from what you fear. Don't you feel relieved and less anxious when you do this?

Unfortunately, not only does avoiding fearful situations appear sensible, it seems to work.

In the short-term, avoidance and escape give you a sense of control over your anxiety.
The problem is that in the long-term you spend more and more time organising your life to avoid what you fear. Fear spreads throughout your life.

HOW PHOBIAS GROW
Phobic avoidance develops a little like a child's tantrum to get something to eat when out shopping. Supermarkets are designed so that the aisle containing the lollies is far enough

don't panic   **39** from the entrance for children to have had time to get tired and hungry. When the lollies finally come into view, the child throws a tantrum.

To a frustrated parent, the lollies provide a simple solution to stop the noise and embarrassment. The problem is that the next time the parent ventures into the supermarket, a tantrum is even more likely.

Avoiding or escaping from what you fear is like giving a kid a lolly to stop a tantrum. Every time that you enter an anxious situation and

> **Avoiding or escaping from what you fear is like giving a kid a lolly to stop a tantrum.**

leave before your anxiety subsides, you make it more likely that you will be anxious next time.

Look what happened to Samantha, who had a phobia about lifts.

"I had decided to catch a lift to the first floor. I approached the lift feeling very anxious. My heart was pounding so hard I thought it might burst through my chest. I was sweating and shaking. I felt lightheaded, my mouth was dry, and I was breathless.

"As I pressed the button, my anxiety shot up. I had an overwhelming desire to go home. I waited for an eternity, my legs became weak and I thought I might collapse. When the lift doors opened, my anxiety rose to a level I previously thought impossible. I turned and ran, immediately feeling immense relief, and vowed never to enter a lift again."

That experience of relief "rewarded" Samantha's anxiety, in the same way that tantrums are rewarded with lollies. Each time you turn anxiety off by escaping, it actually gets stronger. If you continually avoid and escape, anxiety only grows.

CONTROLLING ANXIETY BY FACING YOUR FEARS

To master your anxiety, you have to face your fears. This should be done gradually, controlling your anxiety with slow breathing at every step. By facing your fears gradually your anxiety will not go beyond moderate, manageable levels, and you will be able to endure it until it decreases. If you flee from what you fear while anxiety is rising, it will be rewarded and strengthened. If you wait until it has decreased the anxiety will not be rewarded and it will be weakened.

FACT FILE

Summary
• *Avoiding and escaping increases future anxiety.*
• *Gradually facing your fears, while controlling anxiety, decreases future anxiety.*

The most common mistake made by people trying to manage fears is to progress too quickly. Their anxiety reaches very high levels and never subsides until they run away from the frightening situation.

This can be quite demoralising, and that's why you should face your fears gradually. More about this in the following chapter

don't panic

CHAPTER 6

GAINING CONTROL BY FACING FEARS

To face your fears in an orderly way, you first must clearly identify what you want to achieve. Your goal may be to go somewhere or do something that you presently find frightening. Remember, a goal is something to strive towards; don't worry if you can't achieve it yet – this chapter will explain how you'll be able to break it down into easier, manageable steps.

It is important to make your goals as specific as possible.

A goal is specific when you can answer "yes" to the question: "Could anyone read what I want to do, and do exactly the same task?"

WHAT DO YOU FEAR AND AVOID?

Write down a list of the goals you would like to be able to achieve.

- Make sure that someone could read each goal and do exactly the same task.
- Use the table opposite as an example.
- When you have worked out your goals, rank them in terms of their difficulty.

Give the easiest goal the number 1 (because you will work on this first); the next easiest goal the number 2 (because you will work on this goal second); and so on, until all of your goals are numbered.

don't panic

GOALS	RANK
1.	
2.	
3.	
4.	
5.	
6.	
7.	
8.	
9.	
10.	

BREAKING DOWN YOUR GOALS

To achieve your goals, you have to break them into smaller, easier steps. Once again, each step must be specific. In order to work out your own

don't panic

steps, it may help to read about goals and the "stepladders" that were developed by others to cope with their fears.

Elizabeth's story

Elizabeth had social anxiety disorder. She defined her goal as "to speak in public". However, she decided that this goal was not specific enough, and so she decided to work towards giving a two-minute speech at Toastmasters.

Here's how Elizabeth broke down her task.

- Goal: Give a two-minute speech at Toastmasters
- Step 1: Ask a stranger for directions
- Step 2: Speak with my neighbour for two minutes
- Step 3: Practise a prepared speech in front of a mirror
- Step 4: Join Toastmasters and listen to five speeches
- Step 5: Give a one-minute speech at Toastmasters
- Step 6: Give a two-minute speech at Toastmasters

Elizabeth was then able to say that someone else could read her goal and do exactly the same exercise.

Jonathan's story

Jonathan feared travelling in lifts. He developed the following steps.

- Goal: Travel 50 floors in an express lift
- Step 1: Walk to a lift and push the button
- Step 2: Get inside an empty lift for one minute while a friend keeps the doors open

- Step 3: Get inside an empty lift alone keeping the doors open for one minute
- Step 4: Travel in a glass lift, one floor
- Step 5: Travel in an enclosed lift, two floors
- Step 6: Travel in an enclosed lift, five floors
- Step 7: Travel in an enclosed lift, 10 floors
- Step 8: Travel in an express lift, 20 floors
- Step 9: Travel in an express lift, 50 floors

Sheila's story

Sheila continually visited her doctor, fearing that the nausea she felt after eating must mean that she had stomach cancer. She developed the following steps to deal with her fear.

- Goal: Eat a two-course meal and not see a doctor for one week afterwards
- Step 1: Drink a can of drink outside the hospital. Do not visit the doctor until the next morning
- Step 2: Drink a can of drink at home. Do not visit a doctor for two days
- Step 3: Eat one cracker biscuit outside the doctor's surgery. Do not visit the doctor for three days
- Step 4: Eat a sandwich at home. Do not visit the doctor for four days
- Step 5: Eat a sandwich and dessert at home. Do not visit the doctor for five days
- Step 6: Eat a two-course meal at home. Do not visit the doctor for one week

Ashley's story

Ashley feared her heart pounding because she thought this meant she was about to die of a heart attack, and so tended to avoid physical activity. Realising that this was not healthy or desirable, she worked out the following exercise to face her internal bodily fears.

- Goal: Run vigorously for 20 minutes
- Step 1: Walk up and down stairs for five minutes
- Step 2: Walk up and down stairs for 10 minutes
- Step 3: Run up and down stairs for five minutes, fast enough to feel the heart pounding
- Step 4: Run up and down stairs for 10 minutes, fast enough to feel the heart pounding
- Step 5: Run vigorously for 20 minutes

ACHIEVING YOUR GOALS, STEP BY STEP

Take the goal that you gave the number 1 and develop five or six steps to achieve that goal.

If you need more steps, break the goal down into sub-goals.

If you can achieve the goal in one step, develop a new, more difficult goal that can be broken down into smaller steps.

Use the chart below as an example.

IDENTIFY ALL OF YOUR GOALS – THEN WORK OUT HOW YOU'LL ACHIEVE THEM

GOAL 1

Step 1

Step 2

Step 3

Step 4

Step 5

Step 6

Now work through the same steps for your second goal. Later you can work through your remaining goals.

GOAL 2

Step 1

Step 2

Step 3

Step 4

Step 5

Step 6

FACING YOUR FEARS

Begin with your first goal. Once you have achieved this goal, move on to your second. Progress this way until you have achieved all of your goals. The key to success is gradual but regular progress. While doing so, you may wish to bear some guidelines in mind:

- Use slow breathing before you attempt each step.
- Do not smoke or drink coffee before you attempt each step.
- Never leave because of fear. Only go after your anxiety has begun to decline.
- Expect to feel panicky; use slow breathing to control it.

> **Face your fears regularly. If you leave long gaps your confidence will weaken.**

- Repeat each step until anxiety has decreased and your confidence has increased enough for you to attempt the next step. However, do not be over-cautious. The worst that can happen if you attempt a step before you are ready is that you will become panicky. You will then have to work hard with your slow breathing to keep control.
- Face your fears regularly. If you leave long gaps you will find that your confidence to control your anxiety weakens.
- Reward yourself. No one else understands how frightening your steps are for you, so they can't be expected to congratulate you. So praise yourself or give yourself a treat whenever you face your fear and your anxiety decreases.

A WORD OF CAUTION

People with anxiety problems have many ways of avoiding their fears. Some strategies are obvious, but many are quite subtle.

Look through the following list and see if you use any of the strategies to minimise anxiety, or avoid having to confront your fears.

- Avoiding or escaping from feared situations
- Avoiding exercise or hot/humid conditions
- Having a tablet with you "just in case"
- Asking others to do feared tasks for you
- Drinking alcohol
- Taking too many drugs or medications
- Thinking of something else
- Getting someone to distract you
- Playing loud music
- Keeping silent
- Checking, counting or washing
- Avoiding social contact
- Seeking reassurance
- Thinking of something "good"
- Eating or drinking

These and any other avoidances will need to be overcome. It is not that avoidances do not help in the short-term. It is just that in

Avoid 'avoidances'. They may help in the short-term, but they won't control fear.

the long-term, they do not help you to control your fear.

Take distraction, as an example. Every time you become anxious and distract yourself the anxiety decreases. It rewards anxiety and tells you that next time you become anxious to distract yourself. The problem is that distraction does not modify the core element of your fear. It leaves you feeling just as incapable of controlling panic in the future. Subtle avoidances like distraction, while not harmful, are not helpful because they do not allow you to gain mastery over anxiety.

FACT FILE

Summary
- *Facing your fears is frightening, but when you do, you begin to master your anxiety.*
- *Anxiety, which eventually declines when you face your fears, signals progress.*
- *Never leave because of fear.*
- *Use the slow breathing technique to control anxiety.*

AM I GETTING WORSE?

When you start to face your fears, you feel as though you are getting worse. Your anxiety feels stronger and your ability to control it weaker. This experience is not only normal, it is a signal that you are beating your anxiety. Your anxiety is behaving like the child in the supermarket who screams to get a lolly. The more you say "No", the louder your anxiety will scream to make you give in. Expect a tantrum – and use all of your resources to manage it without avoiding or escaping.

CHAPTER 7

ALL ABOUT WORRY AND OBSESSIONS

People with anxiety problems worry. Sometimes their worry and obsessions are directed inwards, about possible physical or mental illness. At other times, the worry and obsessions are directed outwards, about possible unpleasant events happening to you or others, such as fears of particular objects or situation, financial difficulties, and so on. Although the subject of worries varies, all worry makes anxiety worse.

HOW WORRY WORSENS ANXIETY

When faced with a threat, we think: "Is this dangerous and where is safety?" This reaction is a normal part of the flight or fight response that protects us from danger.

When these thoughts occur as part of a true alarm, there is no problem. When worrying thoughts occur as part of a false alarm, the result is quite different.

When there is no danger, you find yourself in the vicious circle we discussed in Chapter 3. The more you worry, the more anxious you become. The more anxious you become, the more you worry. Some people do things to cope with worry.

Trying to cope by doing things like washing, checking, and seeking reassurance may help in the short-term, but in the long-term this only helps worry and obsessions to grow.

The diversity of worries makes it difficult to list such thoughts. Indeed, the better your imagination, the more things you will find to worry about. Here are some common ones – the trigger first, followed by the accompanying worrying thought.

TYPICAL TRIGGERS AND WORRYING THOUGHTS

- Heart pounding or chest pain
  What if I'm having a heart attack?
- Dizziness
  What if I pass out?
- Things feel unreal
  What if I'm going crazy?
- Urge to flee
  What if I hurt someone or draw attention to myself?
- Shaking
  What if others see me?
- Looking nervous
  What if other think badly of me?
- Blushing
  What if everyone knows I am scared?
- "Jelly legs"
  What if I collapse?
- Bodily pain
  What if I have a serious disease?
- Urge to urinate
  What if I wet myself in public?
- Being in public
  What if other people are watching me?
- Repeatedly feeling anxious
  What if this stress eventually kills me?
- Breathlessness
  What if I suffocate and die?

- Feeling anxious
  What if this stress rises forever and overwhelms me?
- Choking
  What if I vomit over everyone around me?
- Lightheadedness
  What if I'm having a stroke?
- Desire to escape
  What if I lose control?
- Sweating
  What if everyone sees my anxiety?
- Watching the news
  What if a disaster happens to my family?
- Trembling
  What if people think I'm a drug addict?
- Feeling dirty
  What if I get a disease?
- Seeing an electrical switch
  What if it's faulty and the house burns down?
- Bizarre thoughts
  What if no one else has thoughts like these? I must be mad or wicked to have such crazy thoughts.

SOLVING PROBLEMS BY STRAIGHT THINKING

If worry makes anxiety worse, what is the solution? Put simply, it is necessary to think straight and solve any problems as they arise. Although easier said than done, this is not impossible.

If you try to challenge worrying thoughts when you are anxious your mind will jump from worry to worry and you will not be able to think straight. So you should practise thinking through worries when you are calm. Let's look at some examples of how to do this.

don't panic

Eric's story

Eric worried that his pounding heart would eventually cause a heart attack and he would die.

He found it more helpful to think: "My doctor has checked me out and I've had many medical tests, all of which have shown that my heart is in excellent shape. My heart is pumping fast

> **The more you worry, the faster your heart beats. Think it's OK, and it will slow down.**

because my body needs more oxygen. The more I worry about my heart pounding, the faster it will beat. If I start believing my heart is OK, it will eventually slow down."

Eric's primary strategy in tackling worry was to ask himself, "What is the evidence for what I thought?" He found that there was no evidence that he was having a heart attack, but there was evidence that he was anxious.

Eric used a second strategy, which was to ask himself, "What is the effect of thinking the way I do?" Eric wanted his heart to slow down, so he asked himself if his worrying helped him to achieve this.

He decided it did not, and so chose another, more relaxing thought which did slow his heart.

Mary's story

Mary's problem was that when she became anxious, things around her seemed "unreal", which made her worry that she was about to lose control and go mad.

She found it more helpful to think, "I have a sense of unreality because I am overbreathing. If I slow my breathing, these feelings will pass.

don't panic

I am not going mad because overbreathing does not cause insanity. I have had these feelings before and I did not lose control; there is no reason to believe this time will be different. My anxiety may feel out of control but I have never acted out of control before. The sooner I slow my breathing, the sooner I will feel less anxious and more in control."

FACT FILE

Summary
There are three strategies for challenging worrying thoughts and thinking straight. They involve asking yourself:

1. What is the evidence for what I thought?

2. What is the effect of thinking the way I do?

3. What alternatives are there to what I thought?

Like Eric, Mary looked for evidence to support her worries, and found none. She also asked herself, "What alternatives are there to what I thought?" At first she thought that feeling "unreal" must signal insanity.

As an alternative to this way of thinking, she identified her sensations as anxiety made worse by overbreathing. This realisation helped her to stop her anxiety spiralling into panic.

More about straight thinking next chapter.

CHAPTER 8

HOW TO STOP WORRY
BY THINKING STRAIGHT

Worrying thoughts drive the vicious circle of anxiety. With every worrying thought, anxiety rises a little more. In the last chapter we saw that worrying thoughts can be challenged. Challenging such thoughts enables you to jump out of the vicious circle and stop anxiety rising.

As we've seen, worrying thoughts can be challenged with three questions:

- What is the evidence for what I thought?
- What is the effect of thinking the way I do?
- What alternatives are there to what I thought?

Before challenging your own worries with these three questions, practise working through the following examples.

Challenge each worry by writing a more helpful response in the space provided. (Use a separate sheet of paper if you need more space.)

After you have written your answers, compare them with the possible responses on page 58.

Practice 1
When I get anxious I shake so much that
everyone can see. People will see me trembling
and think I am strange.

Practice 2
I can't stand the way I am feeling. What if I am
like this for the rest of my life?

Practice 3
What if the medical tests have been wrong and
there is something wrong with me? I may only
have weeks to live.

Practice 4
What if my anxiety were to rise into panic?
Something terrible would happen. I don't know
what, but something bad would occur.

POSSIBLE RESPONSES

Now that you've worked through these four practice exercises, you may find it helpful to compare your responses with the various possibilities that follow.

Possible response to Practice 1

- What is the evidence for what I thought?
  When anxious I feel as if I am shaking in a very obvious way, but most of the time people do not even know I am anxious.
- What alternatives are there to my thoughts?
  Even if people noticed me trembling they would not think I was strange; at worst they would think I'm tense. Anxiety is a normal emotion so they would not think that I was odd just because I'm anxious.

Possible response to Practice 2

- What is the effect of my thinking?
  As long as I do not work to control my anxiety I will stay this way. The harder I work, the sooner I will be in control.

Possible response to Practice 3

- What is the evidence for what I thought?
  My symptoms are easily explained in terms of anxiety and overbreathing, not as a physical or mental disease.
- What is the effect of my thoughts?
  One day I will only have weeks to live, but if I spend my life worrying about that time I will have a terrible life.
- What alternatives are there to my thoughts?
  Even if the tests are wrong, I will overcome my anxiety and live unrestricted by fear.

Possible response to Practice 4
- What alternatives are there to my thoughts?
  What is the evidence for what I thought?
  In the past, my anxiety always decreased and
  there is no reason to believe that this time
  will be different.
- What is the effect of my thoughts?
  The more I worry about my anxiety,
  the longer it will last. Just because I am
  anxious, danger is not more likely. It is just
  that my flight or fight response is working
  well and looking for danger.

IDENTIFYING THINKING ERRORS

Now that you've practised challenging worrying
thoughts you can extend your skills. Worrying
thoughts can be categorised into thinking errors.
With practice you'll be able to identify each
thinking error when you're anxious.

It then becomes easier to challenge
worries because you'll know the problem that
you're dealing with.

Work through each of the following practice
examples. This time no answers are provided.

To check your answer, ask yourself:

"If I had this worrying thought, would I
believe my challenge? Would believing the new
thought ease my anxiety?" If you answer "no",
you will need to try again.

Thinking error 1
- *Black and white thinking*
  In this way of thinking, things are either
  safe or dangerous – there is no middle
  ground. An example of this type of thinking:
  "I know what I fear is very dangerous."

Thinking error 2

- *Using absolute terms*
  Beware of words like always, never,
  everyone, no one, everything, or nothing.
  Is any situation really that clear-cut?
  An example: "I'll never make any progress in
  controlling my fears."

Thinking error 3

- *Condemning yourself*
  Don't label yourself a failure or worthless
  because of a single mistake or problem.
  An example: "Why am I afraid in situations
  where other people remain calm? I'm
  useless!" Continually putting yourself down
  erodes your self-confidence and cuts off
  the possibility of change. Try to think in
  ways that encourage you to work towards
  controlling your fears.

Thinking error 4

- *Concentrating on weaknesses and
  forgetting strengths*
  An example of this thinking error: "I caught
  the lift one floor, but I could never travel
  two floors." Think of times you have tried or
  even succeeded at something. Consider
  the resources that you really have.

Thinking error 5

- *Overestimating the chances of disaster*
  An example: "I could never speak in public
  because people would think I was boring
  and leave." Things do go wrong from time
  to time, but are you overestimating
  the possible dangers of your situation?

Thinking error 6

- *Exaggerating the important of events*
  An example of this thinking error: "My
  breathing rate is not decreasing fast enough
  and I have been practising for two weeks
  now." Often we think that something is
  more important than it turns out to be.
  Ask yourself: "What difference will it
  make in a week or 10 years?"

Thinking error 7

- *Fretting about how things ought to be*
  Saying that things "should" be different, or
  that you "must" act in a certain way,
  indicates that you may be worrying about
  how things "ought" to be rather than
  dealing with them as they are. An example:
  "I should not be so tense. There must be
  something wrong with my brain chemistry."

Thinking error 8

- *Predicting the future*
  An example of this thinking error: "I have
  had fears for years. I will always be afraid."
  Just because you acted a certain way in
  the past does not mean you have to act
  that way for ever.

CHALLENGING YOUR WORRIES

You can use straight thinking to challenge any
worrying thoughts and recognise any thinking
errors. You may find that just thinking about
your worries makes you anxious.

This is normal and you can even use straight
thinking to tackle this difficulty. You may say to
yourself, "Thinking about my fears does not make

Adrian, who had social anxiety disorder,
thought the following:

Description of Situation	Worrying Thoughts and Old Anxiety Rating	Helpful Thoughts and New Anxiety Rating
Drinking coffee in front of people	Oh no! I might shake and spill the coffee. They will see me shaking and they will think I am mad. They won't like me and they'll move away or turn away. They might even talk about me. That would be awful because I can't stand to appear conspicuous, or tense, or nervous, because other people will think that I'm a failure.	I probably won't spill the drink as I usually cope OK. They may see me, but they probably won't notice me. They probably wouldn't think anything of it. Even if they did, they would probably think that I'm tense or ill. They won't talk about me as they have much more interesting things on their minds.
	Anxiety 80/100	Anxiety 45/100

them more likely to happen. Although I become anxious when I consider my fears, my anxiety will decrease as I develop helpful ways of thinking about my anxiety."

Use the exercise on page 64 to challenge your worries. To help you we have provided an example in the box opposite.

THE IMPORTANCE OF BELIEVING YOUR THOUGHTS

Remember, there is no point in writing "helpful" thoughts that you don't really believe and that only increase your anxiety.

For instance, Wendy forgot her shopping list and worried, "What if I am getting Alzheimer's disease?" She challenged this fear with the thought: "Only one in 10 people my age get Alzheimer's disease." This "helpful" thought did

Make sure the thoughts with which you challenge unhelpful beliefs are realistic.

not decrease her anxiety because she then thought: "I must be the one in 10."

Realising her mistake, she told herself, "I forget things when I am anxious. Right now I feel hot, sweaty, nervous and shaky. It is more likely that I forgot the shopping list because I am anxious." She believed this thought and so her anxiety decreased. So make sure that the thoughts with which you challenge unhelpful beliefs are convincing and realistic.

FACING YOUR FEARS

Perhaps the best way to believe your new thoughts is to put your faith to the test. Facing your fears is the way to do this. We have talked

don't panic

Fill in your own examples here, or use a separate sheet of paper following this example.

Description of Situation	Worrying Thoughts and Old Anxiety Rating	Helpful Thoughts and New Anxiety Rating
	Anxiety /100	Anxiety /100

about this in Chapter 6 and you can practise
your new skills of challenging unhelpful thoughts
as you face your fears. Each time you face
a fear you will become more confident that
the outcomes you worried about are not as bad
or as likely as you had thought.

SOLVING PROBLEMS WITH A STRUCTURED APPROACH

While facing fears and straight thinking can
reduce some worries and obsessions, other
worries need a systematic strategy to solve them.
This involves breaking the problem-solving
process down into a number of tasks.

One structured approach to solving problems,
which research has shown to be very effective,
involves the following steps:

1. Identify the problem

Realising that you have a problem is one thing,
correctly identifying it is another. You may know
that something is wrong with your car because it
makes strange noises, but knowing what part to
replace requires careful thought and diagnosis.

Whenever you have difficulties, write down
what the problem really is (not what tells you
that you have a problem).

For instance, financial difficulties may
signal that something is wrong. They are not
the problem so much as a symptom of the real
problem – poor budgeting or a low-paying job.

2. Brainstorm solutions

Write down as many solutions as possible. Do
not try to keep them in your head because this
will probably only cause confusion.

don't panic

ALL ABOUT
TENSION

The flight or fight response involves increased muscle tension, so it's not surprising that your muscles tighten when you are worried or panicky. However, if physical tension remains too high for too long, it leaves you exhausted and in pain. To overcome problem tension it is necessary to:

- Recognise excess tension
- Relax excess tension away
- Keep excess tension away

Managing physical tension is critical to managing anxiety. When you are tense, your flight or fight response is activated and panicky false alarms are likely. You breathe faster and overbreathing is more likely. Your mind becomes more alert, and intrusive, worrying thoughts may trouble you. All of this means that a high level of background tension increases anxiety.

GOOD AND BAD TENSION

The first step in recognising excessive tension is distinguishing between good and bad tension.

The difference is clearly seen in a game of tennis. Immediately before a serve, players tense up. Their muscles tighten so they are ready to leap into action when the ball is served. They remain tense until the point is over and then they relax. Throughout the game the players

Body area	Where am I tense right now?	Where am I usually tense?
Neck and head • Neck • Scalp • Forehead • Eyes • Temples • Jaw		
Upper body • Shoulders • Top of back • Chest		
Hands and arms • Hands • Lower arms • Upper arms		
Lower body • Stomach • Base of back • Buttocks • Groin		
Legs • Thighs • Knees • Calves • Feet		

don't panic

alternate between being tense and relaxed. Obviously, if the players remained too tense between points they would tire themselves out.

On the other hand, if they relaxed when playing they would not play their best. Their

> **Tension should not be too high for the task, and should last only as long as it needs to.**

tension is good tension because it is not too high for the task and it lasts as long it needs to.

In the same way, you need to be more and less tense throughout the day.

It is necessary to be tenser while driving a car than, for example, when watching television. The tension increases mental alertness that is necessary for driving. The same degree of alertness is not required for watching television.

Tension becomes a problem when muscles remain highly activated. People often tense their shoulders while sitting, squeeze a pen tightly while writing, clench their fists while talking, or tighten their jaws while driving.

In each case the tension is not necessary for the task at hand, and it often continues long after the activity has finished.

WHERE IS YOUR EXCESS TENSION?
Ask yourself where you feel tense right now and then where you usually feel tense. On the table on page 69, put a tick against every area that is relaxed. Put a cross against every area that is tense. Leave blank any area that is neither tense nor relaxed.

See if your tense and relaxed areas tend to group together. You may be very tense around

don't panic

the shoulders and neck, or in the legs. Write down where your tension appears highest and where you are most relaxed.

Where I am usually most tense	Where I am usually most relaxed

You now have a list of areas that are usually tense and relaxed. The relaxed areas are your strong points. The tense areas are your trouble spots where you will have to target your relaxation. In the next chapter, we'll look at whole relaxation – learning how to relax every muscle in your body.

FACT FILE

Summary
• *Tension is bad when it is too high or held for too long.*
• *Recognising excess tension is the first step towards relaxation.*

CHAPTER 10

CONTROL TENSION BY MUSCLE RELAXATION

Now that you've located your excess tension, the good news is that you can remove it by learning the art of muscle relaxation. You can conquer tension with relaxation because the two processes work against each other.

The more tense you become, the less relaxed you are. The more relaxed you become, the less tense you are.

Both the flight or fight response and

If you load your personal scales with relaxation, you will have less tension.

the relaxation response are controlled by the involuntary nervous system.

One half of the involuntary nervous system triggers flight or fight, while the other half controls the relaxation response.

These two halves work like a pair of scales. If you load one side of the scales with panic, worry and overbreathing, you will have more tension than relaxation (because you have fed the flight or fight response).

If you load the other side with slow breathing, straight thinking and relaxation, you will have more relaxation than tension (because you have fed the relaxation response).

Try to relax the muscles around your eyes. You may find that relaxing these muscles is not so easy. You are probably able to direct your attention towards your eyes but may have difficulty knowing how to relax the muscles.

Try another way. Close your eyes tightly. You are now taking control of your muscles, making them do what you want. Once this tension is under control, relax the muscles by opening your eyes.

Alternating tensing and relaxing in this way highlights the two principles of physical relaxation. First: the muscles are deliberately tensed to take control of tension. The idea is not to increase physical tension, but simply to tighten the muscles sufficiently for you to recognise physical tension. Second: the muscles are then relaxed.

You can progressively work through your body, gently tensing and relaxing all your muscles in turn. In this way you can totally relax your whole body. Let's start by learning how to identify and relax each muscle area.

FACT FILE

The benefits of relaxation
When the scales are tipped towards flight or fight you become apprehensive and false anxiety alarms may be triggered. Physical tension brings discomfort and exhaustion. You may become keyed up, on edge, irritable and easily fatigued. You may also experience headaches, backaches, sore muscles, nausea, stomach upsets and "butterflies", and have trouble sleeping.

Removing tension brings comfort and vitality. To achieve relaxation, you have to be able to recognise the signs of physical tension and learn how to control them. This is done by something called progressive muscle relaxation. This chapter explains how to do this so that you can achieve mastery over your own body and anxiety symptoms.

RELAXING EACH MUSCLE GROUP

• Hands. To tense your hands, curl them into fists. To relax them, stop making a fist.

• Lower arms. Tense your lower arm muscles by lowering your hand. Bend it down at the wrist as though trying to touch the underside of your arm. You should feel the tension in your forearm. Relax the muscles by straightening the wrist again.

• Upper arms. Tense your biceps by bending your arm at the elbow, curling your hand towards your shoulder. This is the same movement that bodybuilders use to show off their biceps. Relax the arm by straightening it.

Alternately tensing and relaxing highlights the two principles of physical relaxation.

• Shoulders. Tense the muscles by lifting your shoulders. Hunch them up as if trying to cover your ears with them. Now relax by letting your shoulders drop again.

• Neck. Lean your head to the left until you feel the muscles tighten in the right side of your neck. Slowly and carefully roll your head forward, around to the right and then all the way back to where you started.
One side of the neck will tense while the other is relaxing. If you feel any pain, you are stretching too vigorously.

• Forehead and scalp. Tense the muscles by raising your eyebrows. Release the tension by allowing your face to resume its normal expression once more.

• Eyes. Tense the muscles around the eyes, hold, and then relax.

- Jaw. Tense the jaw by clenching your teeth (enough to tighten the muscles and no more). Relax by unclenching them.
- Chest. Inflate your lungs to expand and tense your chest muscles. Hold the tension, then release by breathing out.
- Stomach. Push your tummy out to tense your stomach muscles. Release by letting your stomach return to its normal position.
- Upper back. Tighten the muscles by pulling your shoulders forward while leaving your arms by your sides. To relax, let your shoulders swing back to their usual position.
- Lower back. While sitting, arch your lower back by dropping your head forward. Your back should roll into a smooth arc, tensing the lower back as you lean forward. Now relax the muscles by sitting up straight again.
- Buttocks. Tighten your buttocks by pulling them together. You'll rise in your chair. Release the tension by sinking back into it.
- Thighs. While sitting, push your feet firmly into the floor to tighten your thigh muscles. Relax by stopping pushing.
- Calves. Lift your toes towards your shins to tighten your calf muscles. Now release the tension by dropping your toes again.
- Feet. Curl your toes down so that they are pressing against the floor. Now release by letting them straighten back to their normal position.

WHOLE BODY RELAXATION

Now that you have practised each exercise, try doing them all in turn to relax your whole body. It is best to do these exercises while sitting in a comfortable but straight-backed chair, with

don't panic

your feel flat on the floor and hands resting in your lap. Sitting is preferable to lying down, otherwise the urge to sleep may become overwhelming. Allow yourself around 15-20 minutes in which you will not be disturbed. You may like to play soothing music, dim the lights, and draw the curtains.

Now close your eyes and get to work. The exercises should begin with the hands, moving up the arms, through the shoulders to the head

> **Close your eyes and get to work. Begin with your hands and move on through the body.**

and then down through the chest and back, finally moving down through the buttocks and legs to the feet. If necessary, leave this book open beside you to remind you of these exercises; with practice, you will soon be able to complete the whole series without the book.

Your body has a natural rhythm. As you breathe in, you tend to tense. As you breathe out, you tend to relax. For this reason it is easiest to breathe in as you tense your muscles and breathe out as you release the tension.

As you work through each of the muscle groups, try to:
- Apply enough pressure to feel tension (as you breathe in)
- Hold tension for 7-10 seconds
- Let the tension go (as you breathe out)
- Wait 10 seconds
- Apply tension again or move on.

When you have finished relaxing, you will probably want to remain seated for a few minutes to enjoy the pleasant feeling. Try not to

don't panic

jump up too quickly as you may tense up again; you may even feel dizzy, as your blood pressure drops when you relax.

You should also be aware your mind becomes less focused when your relax, and tends to wander. Recognise this sign of relaxation and gently bring your mind back to the exercises.

Bear in mind that physical relaxation is an art that takes persistence to master. Only a few people enjoy their first attempt; it is only with patient practice over a two-month period that relaxation becomes a useful strategy in managing excess tension.

More often, people find the bodily sensations of relaxation unusual and possibly worrying: many feel lightheaded, or notice their heart beating. Whatever sensations you have, it is important that you label them as part of the relaxation process. With practice, you'll learn that the sensations aren't frightening and they become less noticeable over time.

QUICK RELAXATION
One of the primary benefits of whole body relaxation is that you learn to recognise excess tension and replace it with relaxation. However,

Learn and practise the quick relaxation method. It can be adapted to any situation.

whole body relaxation is time-consuming and it's not always possible to find the 20 minutes you will need to relax totally. When time is short, you can modify the normal progressive relaxation to a quick relaxation program. Quick relaxation can be adapted to any situation. Although it may not bring the same degree of relaxation as the full 20 minutes of progressive muscle relaxation, it can be targeted at particular muscles. To relax quickly you need to:

- Identify which muscles are too tense
- Tense those muscles (as you breathe in) for 7-10 seconds
- Allow the muscles to relax (as you breathe out) for 7-10 seconds

HOW TO STAY RELAXED

Whole body and quick muscle relaxation can be combined to tackle physical tension. When you know that a difficult day lies ahead, you may prepare yourself by progressively relaxing your whole body at the outset and then by using quick relaxation to stay relaxed.

If you are facing your fears, it is helpful to relax your whole body before you begin the next step in working towards your goal. In this way you will be more relaxed before you confront what lies ahead. Then you can use quick muscle relaxation to remain relaxed while you face and overcome your fears.

FACT FILE

Summary

- *The relaxation response is opposite to the flight or fight response.*
- *Whole body muscle relaxation is useful for relaxing in a general, total sense, especially before stressful activities.*
- *Quick relaxation is useful for keeping muscles relaxed when it is inconvenient to use a whole body relaxation.*

CHAPTER 11

MEDICATION FOR ANXIETY

I f you suffer from "false anxiety alarms" then it is important to reduce the number of times that these false alarms happen. The four-step program of slow breathing, facing fears, relaxation, and worry control will enable you to do this.

An additional way to reduce anxiety alarms is through the use of medication.

In general, anxiety disorders (with the exception of Specific Phobias) can be suppressed with certain medications. Anti-anxiety medications can reduce the frequency and intensity of panic attacks, as well as decreasing levels of general anxiety, tension and worry.

There are many anti-anxiety medications, but broadly speaking they fall into four classes.

Benzodiazepines

A class of medication, such as Valium and Serepax, called the benzodiazepines is specially designed to reduce tension and encourage relaxation, without putting a person to sleep.

These medications work by triggering the brain's own anxiety control mechanisms. They shut down the flight or fight response that we talked about in Chapter 2, meaning that panic and anxiety are less likely to occur. Each member of the benzodiazepines has different strengths

don't panic

and weaknesses and your doctor will be able to work with you to find the most suitable tablet. However, due to their potential addictive qualities, use in the longer-term requires careful medical management.

Tricyclic antidepressants

A second class of anti-anxiety medications, such as imipramine (for example, Tofranil). While they are called "antidepressants" these medications also have specific anti-panic and anti-anxiety qualities. Clomipramine (Anafranil) has also been effective with Obsessive-Compulsive Disorder.

The tricyclic antidepressants have been demonstrated to be effective in treating anxiety disorders (especially panic attacks) and are not addictive. However, they can have side effects, including a dry mouth, dizziness and nausea.

Selective serotonin re-uptake inhibitors

A more recent development in medication for anxiety disorders is the selective serotonin re-uptake inhibitors (SSRIs), such as fluoxetine (Prozac). Like the tricyclics, these drugs have antidepressant qualities, but they also act on the systems in the brain that are involved in fear and anxiety. These medications (for example, sertraline; Zoloft) have the capacity to reduce fear and panic and have fewer side effects than the tricyclic antidepressants.

Other medications

There are a number of other medications that are appropriate with certain anxiety disorders that are not classifiable in the previous groupings. These include buspirone (Buspar), that has been useful in treating Generalised Anxiety Disorder; beta blockers, such as propanalol (Inderal), that have been used in the management of Social Anxiety Disorder; and moclobemide (Aurorix), an antidepressant drug with anti-panic qualities.

DECIDING TO TAKE MEDICATION

The decision to take medication to complement the self-help strategies outlined in this book must be made after careful consultation with your doctor. Here are some questions that you may usefully raise in your discussions.

- *How effective is the medication?*

Ask what percentage of people with your problem improve with the medication you are considering and how this compares with other treatments.

- *What happens when I stop taking it?*

FACT FILE

Summary
- *There are a number of medications for anxiety. Speak with your doctor or psychiatrist about these.*
- *Find the best medication, at the best dose, with the fewest side effects to reduce your false anxiety alarms.*
- *Keep lines of communication with your doctor open.*

Most of these medications discussed relieve anxiety, but it may return soon after the tablets are stopped. Find out how many people relapse, and any other effects that happen at this time.

- *What are the common side effects?*

Side effects vary between people and across different medications. Ask your doctor about these, and if you experience any, discuss these with your doctor, who may consider changing the type of medication or the dose you are taking to help manage any side effects more effectively.

CHAPTER 12

HELPING OTHERS
TO HELP YOU

So far we have been thinking about your problems with anxiety from your point of view. We have been treating the problem as if it is something that you need to confront all by yourself. This can be both good and bad.

It is good because at the end of the day, you are the one who needs to take control of yourself again and stop anxiety and panic controlling you. However, thinking about your anxiety problems only from your point of view overlooks the fact that that you could well have friends

> **Sometimes friends and family, despite their best intentions, can be unhelpful.**

and family who may be helpful in overcoming your anxieties. It also fails to recognise that sometimes our friends and family members can, despite their best intentions, be unhelpful.

Now is a good time to stop and think about how your friends and relatives can be most help-ful. In fact, this chapter is written not for you (a person with an anxiety problem), but for your friends and family members.

You may read it yourself and then talk about the issues with your friends and relatives, or you may find it easier to ask them to read this chapter. Either way, the goal is for you to make sure that those around you are helping and not hindering your progress.

IF YOU KNOW SOMEONE WITH ANXIETY PROBLEMS

"I just wish I had a broken leg, and then people would see there is something wrong with me." It is a common comment of people who suffer from attacks of panic, phobias, uncontrollable tension and worry. Friends and relatives can find it hard to understand how someone cannot cope with anxiety. In fact, everyone seems to be saying, "I know that anxiety is unpleasant. We all get stressed from time to time, but we all get over it sooner or later. So pull yourself together. Enough is enough!"

If you know someone who has an anxiety disorder, then it is not uncommon to feel sympathy at one moment and irritation or despair at another. However, expressing this frustration is not the best way to help.

A better way is to give patient understanding and supportive encouragement.

Patient understanding

To begin with, let's try to foster patient understanding of what it must be like to have an anxiety disorder.

Everyone gets anxious, but not everyone has an anxiety disorder.

We all worry from time to time about our health, family, finances and so on. We all get stressed when the demands of living ask more of us than we can give. However, these are not disorders of anxiety. These are normal

don't panic

experiences that happen to everyone. Indeed, people with anxiety disorders experience many of the same worries, stresses and fears as you.

The chief difference is that someone with an anxiety disorder will say, "I have all those experiences, but this anxiety is different." They have not been able to understand their anxiety

It may be difficult to understand, but don't give up. Ask what their life is like.

disorder in the same way that they understand everyday anxiety. The anxiety disorder feels in a category of its own.

Therefore, if they cannot understand their anxiety disorder in terms of everyday anxiety, then it is probably going to be difficult for you to even try. But don't give up. Instead, ask the person to explain to you what life is like.

Try to put yourself in their shoes. Perhaps you could say, "I know what it is like to be anxious, but that isn't really helping me understand what you are feeling. It seems as if what is happening to you is quite different. Do you think you could help me get some idea of how these anxiety problems are so different from everyday anxiety?" You may find it helpful to read some of the earlier chapters in this book as well.

Being patient
As you come to understand the way that the anxiety disorder affects your friend or relative's life, consider that without treatment, anxiety disorders may last a long time and be very disabling. Although treatments will help, you need to be there for the long haul. Recovery

takes time and you can help by showing that you can see that the person is doing everything they can to cope and to get well. Be patient, because impatience will demoralise.

Supportive encouragement

Once you have begun to understand the anxiety problems, your role can become like a sporting coach. Just as the coach does not play the game, but gives supportive encouragement from the sideline, you can give the continued support and encouragement that your friend or relative needs at each stage.

The hard work of treatment

Recently, there has been much research into the treatment of anxiety disorders. As a result, we know that some medications and a non-drug treatment called "cognitive-behaviour therapy" are effective treatments for anxiety. Cognitive-behaviour therapy aims to change the anxious behaviour and the worrying thoughts (or cognitions) and is the method outlined in this book. It involves many "homework" assignments. These exercises allow the skills to be practised so that real gains can be made. You can help by:
- Giving the person time to practise
- Making some time to ask them how they are going
- Saying "well done!"

Your role is chiefly one of support. Confronting fears can be scary. Therefore, find the right balance between encouraging your friend or relative to face what he or she fears and showing that you're trying to understand how difficult it must be.

don't panic

Medications

If your friend or relative is taking medications to manage anxiety, you can help in remembering to take medications. You may also find it helpful to learn about any side effects. This will help you to respond appropriately. For example, if tiredness is a side effect, then you will know that if the person needs to rest, he or she is not being lazy. Again, if irritability is a side effect, then you may need to be more understanding if there are occasions of short temper.

Maintaining the hard-won gains of treatment

When someone stops taking medications or when he or she finishes the exercises in this book, it will be time to maintain the hard-won gains. It will be advisable to continue confronting previously feared situations, practising relaxation and other anxiety management skills, and ensuring that the thinking is helpful and not anxiety-producing. Providing encouragement to keep going with these activities can help maintain the gains. Progress is not always going to be steady. There will be good days and bad. Throughout these ups and downs you can be a support by encouraging your friend or relative to stick with the treatment that has worked.

FACT FILE

Summary

As a friend or relative of someone who suffers from an anxiety disorder, you can make a valuable contribution to his/her recovery.

By showing patient understanding, you provide them with a trusted person in whom they can confide.

By giving them supportive encouragement, you will be able to balance understanding with assistance in the recovery process.

CHAPTER 13

CHECKING
YOUR PROGRESS

Impatience is a sign of anxiety. So if you have read the book, reached this chapter, and are still looking for "the answer", now is the time to make the four solutions work for you. The only way to master anxiety in the long-term is through patient practice of the techniques discussed.

Practice means working hard every day to master slow breathing, straight thinking and relaxation, while all the time facing your fears. Patience means that you persevere.

Learn the skills and persevere even when you feel as if you will never master the skills. With patient practice you can succeed.

WORDS OF ENCOURAGEMENT

I asked some people who had completed an anxiety management program, similar to the one in this book, what they would have most liked to have known while they were learning to control anxiety. They agreed on five statements:

- Although you feel worse while you face your anxiety, you are actually getting better
- You can control panic, worry and tension with slow breathing, relaxation and straight thinking
- The harder it is to face your fear, the easier it is next time

don't panic

- The biggest gains are made when you confront fears while you feel weakest
- The hard work pays off

FOREWARNED IS FOREARMED

Learning to control your anxiety is possible, but it requires hard work. Yet even for people making excellent progress there are times when managing anxiety seems a hard and unattainable goal. Learning any new skill is difficult.

Mastering anxiety is no different. Expect setbacks to occur, but plan to push through them. Continue controlling your breathing, phobic avoidances, worrying thoughts, and tension and you will be making progress. Progress is difficult when times are tough, but it is at these times when you can make real gains.

During setbacks, keep controlling anxiety. When anxiety is at its most unmanageable, persevere with all of your new skills.

See if you are using every skill and check that you are using them correctly.

Slow breathing
- Are you monitoring your breathing, especially when anxious?
- Are you holding your breath in each slow breathing cycle?
- Are you breathing in a smooth, light way?

Facing your fears
- Are you facing your fears too quickly? If so, slow down to where you are making progress but are still keeping control of anxiety.
- Are you facing your fears too slowly? If so, take the next step in facing your fears. By

don't panic

doing so, you can break the deadlock
when you cannot seem to overcome
a stubborn fear.

- Should you practise some steps more
frequently and for longer?

Straight thinking

- Are you using straight thinking to
manage worries?
- Are you testing your beliefs by facing
your fears?
- Do you believe your helpful thoughts?
- Are you using structured problem solving?

Relaxation

- Are you regularly practising whole
body relaxation, especially before
facing your fears.
- Are you using quick relaxations at the first
sign of anxiety?
- Are you reacting to tension with relaxation?

PERSISTENT WORRIES

After mastering the exercises you may continue
to have worrying thoughts, some of which may
make setbacks more likely.

It is important to avoid saying things such as:
"I'm really hopeless. I'm back where I started."

Instead, it is more helpful to think: "I'm
disappointed that progress is slow and not
plain sailing but I'm not going to turn it into
an excuse for giving up. Instead of being
disappointed, I'll make every effort to progress.
If I keep working, I will master my anxiety."

You may find that you manage anxiety so
well that you stop regular relaxation and slow

breathing. There is nothing wrong with this, you just need to restart implementing the techniques whenever you notice life becoming stressful or if your previous difficulties come back.

Plan to manage such times, rather than to hope they will not occur. However, because anxiety is a normal emotion, it is probable that problem anxiety will re-emerge. But now you can handle problem anxiety differently. You can face your fears in a series of graded steps, thereby reducing phobic fears.

Whole body relaxation can reduce excess tension, and quick relaxation will help maintain the relaxed state. Slow breathing will stop anxiety spiralling into panic, and by thinking straight you can manage worrying thoughts.

Remember, the key to mastery of anxiety is patient practice of all four skills.

CHAPTER 14

WHERE TO SEEK HELP AND ADVICE

Only psychiatrists and other medical doctors can prescribe the anti-anxiety medications described in this book. Many different health professionals can offer psychological treatments for anxiety, however the only psychological therapies with good evidence of long-term efficacy are the ones described in this book. These are called "cognitive behaviour therapies".

Clinical psychologists will be able to help you implement these strategies, but so too can some doctors, psychiatrists, occupational therapists, social workers, and so on.

For help, contact your doctor to find someone who has been trained in cognitive-behavioural treatments for anxiety disorders.

For health professionals interested in training resources relevant to this book, please contact the author for details at:

andrew@psy.uwa.edu.au

USEFUL INTERNET ADDRESSES

Anxiety Network Australia
http://www.anxietynetwork.com.au/

Anxiety Panic Hub
http://www.paems.com.au/index.html

Clinical Research Unit for Anxiety
   and Depression
http://www.crufad.unsw.edu.au/homepage.htm

Social Anxiety Australia
http://www.socialanxiety.com.au/

CLINICS & OTHER USEFUL ADDRESSES

AUSTRALIAN CAPITAL TERRITORY
Building 39, Psychology Clinic, ANU
Canberra, ACT 0200
Tel: (02) 6125 0412   Fax: (02) 6125 9656

NEW SOUTH WALES
Anxiety Disorders Clinic, St Vincent's Hospital,
299 Forbes Street, Darlinghurst, NSW 2010
Tel: (02) 9332 1188 or (02) 9332 1209

Kiloh Centre, Prince of Wales Hospital,
Easy Street, Randwick, NSW 2031
Tel: (02) 9382 4352

Macquarie University Anxiety Research Unit
Department of Psychology
Macquarie University, NSW 2109
Tel: (02) 9850 8711

Macarthur Mental Health Service
6 Browne Street, Campbelltown, NSW 2560
Tel: (02) 4629 5400

Westmead Hospital
Department of Medical Psychology
Westmead, NSW 2145
Tel: (02) 9845 6686

Bankstown Anxiety Clinic
Bankstown-Lidcombe Hospital, Elridge Rd
Bankstown, NSW 2200
Tel: (02) 9722 8992

Nepean Anxiety Disorders Clinic
Clinical Sciences Building, Nepean Hospital
PO Box 63
Penrith, NSW 2751
Tel: (02) 4734 3404

Sydney Anxiety Disorders Practice
28 Harrow Road, Stanmore, NSW 2048
Tel: (02) 9527 0796
Fax: (02) 9557 0174
Website: www.sadp.com.au

Specialty Clinic
Gosford Hospital, 77 Holden Street
Gosford, NSW 2250
Tel: (02) 4320 3242

Anxiety Management Service
Northern Rivers Area Health Service
60 Hunter Street
Lismore, NSW 2480
Tel: (02) 6620 2180

Child & Adolescent Anxiety Clinic
Block 4, Level 2, Royal North Shore Hospital
St Leonards, NSW 2065
Tel: (02) 9926 8905

Child & Adolescent Anxiety Clinic
Macquarie University, NSW 2109
Tel: (02) 9850 8711

NORTHERN TERRITORY
NT Government Mental Health Service
PO Box 40596, Casuarina, NT 0811
Tel: (08) 8999 4988

QUEENSLAND
Obsessive Compulsive Disorder Support Group
20 Balfour Street, New Farm, QLD 4005
(postal address) PO Box 475
Sumner Park, QLD 4074
Tel: (07) 3358 4988

Panic Anxiety Disorders Association (QLD) Inc
PO Box 1405, Stafford, QLD 4053
Tel: (07) 33534851
email: padaqld@bigpond.com

SOUTH AUSTRALIA
Panic Anxiety Disorders Association of SA
PO Box 83, Fullarton, SA 5063
Tel: (08) 8227 1044
Fax: (08) 8227 1266
email: pada@chariot.net.com

Panic Anxiety Education and Management
PO Box 258, Fullarton, SA 5063
Tel: (08) 8555 5012 (also fax)

Obsessive Compulsive Disorder Support (SA)
Tel: (08) 8231 1588

TASMANIA
Tasmanian Association for Mental Health
95-97 Campbell Street,
Hobart, TAS 7000
Tel: (03) 6236 9592

VICTORIA
Panic Anxiety Disorders Association of Victoria
PO Box 186, Burwood, VIC 3125
Tel: (03) 9889 6760
Fax: (03) 9889 1022

Obsessive Compulsive & Anxiety Disorders
   Foundation of Victoria (Inc)
600 Orrong Road
Armadale, VIC 3143
PO Box 358, Mt Waverley, VIC 3149
Tel: (03) 9576 2477 (HelpLine)
Fax :   (03) 9576 2499

WESTERN AUSTRALIA
Robin Winkler Clinic, University of WA
10-12 Parkway, Crawley, WA 6009
Tel: (08) 9380 2644
Fax: (08) 9380 2655

Perth Clinic
29 Havelock Street, West Perth, WA 6005
Tel: (08) 9481 4888
Fax: (08) 9481 4454
Email: info@perthclinic.com.au

Panic Anxiety Disorders Association (WA)
PADAWA at The Niche
Suite B11, Aberdare Road
Nedlands, WA 6009
Tel: (08) 9380 9898
Fax: (08) 9346 7534
Email: padawa@cnswa.au

don't panic